CONTENTS

DEDICATION

◆ ◆ ◆

To Dad for showing me that hard work pays off. <3

To Mom for raising a warrior daughter, even though I was surrounded by brothers and testosterone on every side!

To Dr. Balogun for taking a chance on me and inadvertently changing my life (along with thousands of other nurses' lives by extension) in the process.

And last, but certainly not least…to my amazing husband for 20 years of pure bliss, and for being by my side through this whole crazy journey…here's to 120 more!

MEET MARIE PEPPERS

I always knew I wanted to be a nurse.

Maybe it sounds cliche; maybe you'll think I'm just saying that because it sounds good. But it's not that simple.

I mean, in my day, there weren't many options...if you were female, you became a nurse, a teacher, or a stay at home mother.

And for me, the lure was there from a really young age...I remember being drawn to candy striper uniforms, and feeling the pull to volunteer and save lives.

But my journey into nursing wasn't totally straightforward...is anything in life, really?

My intentions were good; they truly were. But sometimes, even the best-laid plans can be thrown sideways...at least a little bit.

After high school, I made my way to the community college to figure out the prerequisites I needed to become a nurse. But while my heart and mind knew what they wanted, my soul wasn't quite ready.

Let me explain....

Well, there's not much to explain, really. I was young, female, and boy crazy. I just wanted to enjoy life, my youth, to party some more, hang on to what tiny morsel was left of my childhood...call it whatever you like, but yeah, that was the barricade that stood in between myself and starting a career in nursing.

And honestly, I don't see it as a bad thing as I look back. You know as well as I do that nursing is a HARD job...it's hard mentally, emotionally, and physically. And to really do it right, you have to be 100% ready.

So I took the easy route...I went to school to become a medical assistant, and worked for a cardiologist for 3 years. But I regretted not going to nursing school...that was when I knew I was ready. Here's the thing...even when I was boy crazy and too busy having fun to take nursing seriously, I was already inspired to live my life a certain way.

My dad was such a hard worker...he literally worked 2-3 jobs at a time so that my brothers and I (and our mother!) could have the best life ever.

But that's not even what truly inspired me.

My dad didn't just show up and do his job(s). He had his eye on a much bigger prize, and ended up opening a jewelry factory. All of a sudden, he didn't need to work multiple jobs. He got to be home with us for dinner.

I really think that planted the seed in my mind (and heart!) to take everything as far as I can take it...which is what led me to where I am today as a nurse.

Now, let me not deceive you...I didn't just conjure this idea in my head. I'd love to tell you that I did...that I woke up one day and realized that nurses need to have more opportunities to work from home, to be home with their families at dinner time, to actually get to participate in the raising of their children, and most of all, to not have to be on our feet all day for 12 hour shifts... knowing all the while that as soon as this shift is over, we get to go home, sleep, and wake up to do it all over again the next day.

But remember what I said before about the best-laid plans sometimes not panning out the way we thought they would.

Well, in my case, it turned out pretty amazing, and I'm here to help make your career as a nurse turn out the same way, but let me back up a bit and explain how this even came to be.

So, there I was, going about my life as a nurse...and, yeah, I paid my dues, did the long shifts, and all the things that go along with that. So I absolutely DO get what you're going through. And while I've always loved being a nurse, I'm not going to sugarcoat the hell (let's just call it what it is) it is when you're on the floor, trying to take care of seriously ill humans, trying to deal with their sometimes (understandably) hysterical relatives, trying to navigate office politics that have no place in a medical setting, and just trying to stay on your feet for more than 12 hours straight with nary a break to pee when you need to.

I also know that nursing is in our blood. And doing all this is sort of like being a soldier sent out for war...we know we're there to do a very important job.

So I'm not even going to lie...I LOVED my job at the hospital.

BUT....

I saw an advertisement...a blind, confidential one, seeking a dynamic LPN (I couldn't have found better words to describe myself if I tried) to be a trailblazer, forging a new kind of patient connection.

Ummmmm, what?

Yeah, that piqued my interest.

And get this...they only wanted 30 hours a week, flex time...I could do this AND keep my job at the hospital.

No, I wasn't crazy, so please don't ask. I was just adventurous, eager, curious, and VERY inspired by my world-class father.

So, I applied, got a call from the office manager (also known as the doc's wife), and got an invite to an interview for the Care Manager job.

But that wasn't even the best part.

Once she told me the name of the doctor, I had a full-blown nursegasm...he was my parents' doctor, and he'd always taken such great care of them!

My point, and I do have one, is that I already knew that he was an AMAZING internal medicine specialist...I may have been wading into unchartered waters in a rather exciting, "Alice in Wonderland" way, but any fear of the unknown I had dissipated once I learned about the stellar doc guiding me down the rabbit hole.

Turned out that Medicare came out with an amazing new (in 2015) program called Chronic Care Management. And they needed a nurse to lead the way...and I was going to be that nurse.

I wish I could tell you that I'm some kind of genius guru who came up with the idea to create this program to help other nurses make their way into this (no longer new) career path in nursing.

But it all goes back to the best-laid plans, and how they sometimes make their way into your life without your even looking for them.

The truth is that other nurses heard about my new job, and they all wanted in. I didn't have to convince anyone. I didn't have to promote my program. I didn't have to do anything, really, other than putting it together to create an easy to follow course for nurses to change their lives.

And that leads us to today.

So here we are...I've now changed the lives of thousands (soon to be hundreds of thousands!) of nurses with this program. I've expanded it, added new information, and managed to make enough connections to inform the nurses in my private group about every new opportunity that comes up, seeking someone just like them (and like you!) to make a very solid living from the comfort of their (and your!) cozy home office.

And I'm here to tell you that nursing doesn't have to be difficult.

I mean, it's not to say that any nursing job is *easy* because we all know how attached we get to patients, and how much our job affects us even after we're done for the day.

But you don't *need* to be on your feet all day, several days (and nights!) a week to be a nurse who makes a difference in people's lives.

You don't have to go through a hellish commute to get to work in a medical facility where you have to play politics in between just trying to help every person who walks in the door, needing the sort of care that only a nurse can provide.

There's so much more available to you, and it's just as rewarding (if not more so!) without any of the downsides you've come to accept as just part of the job.

So think of this book as an invitation, a personalized one, from me to you. Read on to learn about how I've changed the lives of nurses just like you, and how much happier they are, just for the simple change in their career path that I helped make possible.

I'm not saying this to brag, or toot my own horn. I've no need for pats on the back at this point in my career.

But I want you to see, truly SEE what's possible for you, and how it's closer than you can even begin to imagine.

No, it's not difficult.

No, it's not risky.

No, it doesn't take a long time to get through my course and be totally prepared to interview for a job like this.

No, you don't have to give up what you're doing now in order to do this.

No, there's no catch or drawback.

But don't take my word for it.

Keep reading to hear what other nurses have said about the transformation that happened in their lives...and see how easily YOUR life can change.

Are you ready?

Then turn the page....

DIANA'S STORY

Maybe my story will be the one you remember...because it's not like the others.

How do I know, you ask?

Well, here's the thing...I've been a nurse for over 45 years now. I've done every possible job, from charge nurse, to nurse manager, to floor nurse (and not necessarily in that order!), and I've worked every possible shift. If there's one thing I've learned after talking to too many nurses to even contemplate trying to count, it's that they all seemed to have a "calling," like something within them that led them to become a nurse.

My story isn't like that. For me, there was no calling. In fact, I had no idea whatsoever what I wanted to do with my life.

So let's send a little shoutout to "Golden Girls" because I'm going to tell you my story Sophia-style...ready?

Picture it...some ordinary town, USA, 1972...I was a junior in high school. And there were expectations of me...mainly that I'd be prepared to move on to the next phase of my life with a very clear plan as to what I was going to do with my life.

But I had NO idea. None whatsoever.

Now, this was before computers, social media, and Google. I didn't have the luxury of doing some "research" on the internet. So there I was, sitting in my counselor's office...I still remember Miss Kinch looking at me with a bit of concern, a bit of pity, and perhaps a bit of boredom...this was her work life on repeat...talking to students who had no idea what they wanted to do once they walked across the stage in their caps and gowns.

If you're a young nurse reading this, rest assured, this was NOT the dark ages...we may not have had computers, but believe it or not, there was hope. Miss Kinch gave me a test that I had to fill out with a pencil, old school, and she was going to go through it on her own (as opposed to running it through a computer as it's done today), again...old school.

So I waited. Ok, let me not deceive you. I was young, didn't have a care in the world, and was not too concerned about my future. I mean, I was never actually going to turn the dreaded 30, was I? So I pretty much forgot all about this test.

Until they called me into the counselor's office.

Picture it...chemistry class in Nowheresville, USA...I was called out of class, and all I could think about was what I may have done wrong, and how I was going to convince them that I was totally innocent.

But that was the day my life changed. Because Miss Kinch had some interesting results for me, as far as what I'd excel at in life. There were four options. They were as follows:

- Teacher
- Beautician
- Healthcare related field
- Car Mechanic

Ok, so here's where my brain was that day. I didn't want to get my hands or nails dirty (oh, how little I understood about nursing!), so that ruled out becoming a car mechanic.

And then there were three.

My mother cut my hair, so I didn't know what a beautician was.

And then there were two.

I could have become a teacher, but I actually *enjoyed* the chemistry class I was called out of (yes, really!). I'd always loved science in general.

And then there was one....

So that, ladies and gents, is how I became a nurse. As I said, no calling, no "just knowing," no sense that I *need* to do this. It was just a day in the early 70s when the young version of me, unbeknownst to herself, had made a decision that would change the trajectory of my entire life.

So this is where I started to get my hands dirty...the bulk of my nursing life was spent in cardiology. I'd been a staff nurse, a charge nurse, *that* nurse who teaches patients...I mean, we've talked about this before a bit above, in the earlier part of my story.

But while I may not have had a calling or some kind of invisible homing device that led me to nursing, I sure did take it to heart. I became an Assistant Transplant Coordinator, a Cardiology Manager, and at one point, Director. Telling this part of my story is very heartfelt for me because I participated in the saving of many a life. From heart failure patients who needed a new heart, to those whom we strictly focused on remaining safe and healthy at home (instead of yet another hospital stay). Everything I did, every patient who crossed my path, every new heart that gave another person a new lease on life, well, all of those are forever etched upon *my* heart.

What I'm trying to say is that it doesn't have to be a calling. God made nurses to do His work here on earth. I am certain of it. It's a very special job we do, and no other occupation on the planet quite compares to it.

But there's a dark side of it...what we give with all of our heart, and what we gain from every life that we touch (and that touches us right back), we pay for with our bodies. There is only so much time any human, I don't care how fit or healthy, can manage to stay on his or her feet for 12 (and let's not pretend we actually get to go home after 12 hours, EVER) hours a day (or overnight!). At some point, we're pushed into retirement because we just don't have anything more in us (physically) to give, and it usually starts *way* before actual retirement age.

But we're nurses...we push through it, right? I mean, we've been conditioned to push through anything and everything.

And let's not kid ourselves. We're restless when we're not working and saving lives, too.

So, picture it...there I was, semi-retired, sitting (comfortably!) in my living room, talking to my husband, and that's when it hits me.

"What should I do with all this knowledge in my head?" I asked him, not really expecting any sort of answer. I mean, what could he tell me? All I knew was that it seemed almost sinful to keep all my knowledge that I had to myself, bottled up to muddle around alone in my brain. And that's when the Miss Kinch of my adult life came into my life to forever change my life. Or more accurately, this was the second decision that totally changed the trajectory of my life.

Picture it...my living room, in semi-retirement...I needed a life line. I needed something to do that didn't wear down my already worn down body. I needed to keep saving the world, one patient at a time.

And that's when I found Marie Peppers.

So, here's the thing...nursing may not have started out as a calling in my life, but it surely became one by the time I was having that conversation in my living room with my husband. And maybe my story is one of those where God magically and mysteriously sends the right person into my path to get me onto the right path. The thing about Marie is that she's not like anyone I've ever met before, especially not on social media. She is a true nursing leader. It's as though she sees the problem before it presents itself, and comes up with a solution before you can even process that you have a problem.

What I mean by that is that I didn't see semi-retirement as a problem, per se. One could argue that I've done my duty as a nurse. I could write a whole book about the patients I've helped come out of heart failure and get back into life.

BUT...I wasn't done yet, and I'm still not done. I may be done with the 12 hour shifts, but I'm not done being a nurse, and I don't think I ever will be.

So I was one of the early adopters of Marie's course. And truthfully, I didn't expect much, mainly because I had no idea what to truly expect.

What I did NOT expect was that I'd have a job within two weeks. And that I'd get to continue saving lives as a nurse from the comfort of my living room...that very same living room where a simple question to my husband got this whole party started... but I digress. Get this...I get to work from my sofa, completely comfortable, with zero stress to my body, *and* I get to sip a hot coffee while doing all that.... Every. Single. Day.

I know it may sound bizarre, but I think of Marie as the person who restarted my heart...got me back into life as a nurse, and showed me how powerful I truly am as a nurse, without even having to leave my house.

And let's be honest...with a (seemingly never ending!) pandemic upon us, that is truly a thing of beauty.

But even if we were living in normal times (does such a thing even exist anymore??), how great is that you, too, can be a nurse from the comfort of your living room, saving lives and sipping coffee, without the usual hassles of traffic (is the work commute an enjoyable part of anyone's day?), a grumpy patient, or patient's family member screaming in your face for something that's 100% outside your control.

Yes, you read that right, and it's totally doable. But only with the help of the amazing Marie Peppers. I don't know what you're waiting for, but your new life awaits. Hopefully, once you've taken Marie's course, we can chat about all of this over coffee on our respective sofas. The only regret you'll have is that you didn't meet Marie sooner....

Diana Poorman, RN

ROSEMARY'S STORY

One thing is for certain...nursing is a calling. It's this thing you were born with, that's nestled deep within your soul, and you just know you were born to do this.

Of course, the message is not always clear, straightforward, and direct...sometimes, it's like a dream...the signs are there, the symbolism is deep, but you have to connect the dots yourself.

You're a nurse, so you know the feeling...that deep down desire to serve, to heal, to "fix" things that are broken. Even in old movies where nurses are depicted wearing those ridiculous hats, it's always been a life of service. One could argue that a nurse is the ultimate servant...and you know what they say about servants... a servant is a master in disguise. And when you think about what nurses do...we are the ones who take care of the patients; soothe them, comfort them, and explain things to their worried loved ones. Nurses are, without question, irreplaceable.

I realize I'm getting a bit nostalgic (and perhaps a bit wordy!), but you see, my path to nursing wasn't as direct as most. Let me explain....

You know how they say it takes a village to raise a child?

Well, I was born in a village. Literally. I come from Zimbabwe, Africa.

Yep, you guessed it; I'm a loooong way from home. Except that the

US is my home now. But let's get back to that village for a moment.

I was that village's nanny. And no, I don't mean as a career, or even as a grownup. I was a little kid, caring for babies and other little kids. And the parents trusted me because I was a natural. Simply put, I was born to be a caregiver.

I hadn't put two and two together back then, as in, I hadn't figured out that my purpose in life was to become a nurse. I was too busy enjoying every snuggle with those babies. But life has a way of catching up to you, and at some point, I had to think about my future.

So maybe it sounds cliche, but I made my way to America. And my first thought just as soon as I got here was to take a job as a nanny. We all crave the familiar, especially when you're in a new country that's very far away from the village you grew up in, and I don't just mean in terms of distance. So I took a job with a family that had two young girls, and brought the magic of Africa into their lives. It was an amazing experience.

But familiarity breeds contempt. Soon enough I grew bored, searched for more meaning, and just all around wanted something more. I guess on some level, we're all looking for more, aren't we? But one thing's for certain…we're definitely all looking for meaning in life.

So I took a job as a companion to an elderly woman whose health was failing due to Parkinson's disease. And that's where the seeds of my nursing career truly started to take off…because shortly before that lady died, weak and ravaged by an unforgiving disease as she was, she found a moment of strength to look me in the eye, and tell me that I was made to be a nurse. All I was missing, she stated with as much exuberance as she could muster, was a nursing license.

It was as if the meaning I was so desperately seeking had found me. But life has a way of throwing us curveballs, doesn't it?

Just as I was about to pursue my career in nursing, my daughter Ivy died tragically in a car accident. If you're a nurse (and if you're reading this, you most certainly are) you understand the basics of accidents, and how life is not always fair. If you're a trauma nurse, I imagine you've had to deliver tragic news to many a (rightfully) hysterical and devastated parent. But most of all, if you're a parent, you know that nothing in the world could even begin to compare to the horrors of burying your own child. No amount of tragedy you witness as a nurse can even begin to prepare you.

I'm not going to sugarcoat it. My life fell apart..I was literally bright to my knees. I wanted to die and be with Ivy. Most of all, I needed a reason to *want* to continue living. I mean, let's be honest here…there should be a universal rule that says that parents *always* die before their children; no exceptions.

But sadly, life doesn't work that way, and it's not always forgiving. I had other children who needed me to keep going for them, so if there was ever a moment in my life when I was challenged to keep moving forward, to find a reason (beyond my children) to continue breathing, to find purpose and meaning in my life, this was it. I opened a non-profit in Ivy's name, did a bit of missionary work in my native Africa, and finally took the big leap in becoming a nurse, embracing this new career with both arms, just as I know Ivy would have wanted me to.

My path into nursing is hardly typical, but I must confess that my journey as a nurse was even more unusual. I didn't take a job in a busy medical office, or on a hospital floor. Instead, I went to work in hospice, specifically serving Native Americans on their reservations in New Mexico. It was a beautiful fusion of my own culture delving deep into theirs. Learning about their customs and way of life had a way of making the job all the more meaningful because as you well know, you can't truly be a healer without looking deep into your patient's soul.

My daughter Ivy never left my heart, mind, or spirit, though. They say that time heals all wounds, but I assure you that this isn't true. Time makes the pain a bit duller...it has a way of offering enough distractions to keep going, and if you're lucky enough to find your purpose, it gives you a reason to wake up in the morning. But some wounds never truly heal.

The thing is that I wanted to show up at my very best every day for Ivy because even though we're no longer together in the physical realm, I wanted her to be proud of me. Not just proud because I'm her mother, but proud because I got out of bed on days when I wished I could disappear forever, and showed up for the patients who needed me.

But there's something else I'm certain Ivy did for me.

You know how angels have a way of sending the right people into our lives? I mean, I can't tell you what to believe, but I'm certain that our angels are always looking out for us, and putting everything and everyone we need in our path.

Well, one day, as I was finishing a shift, I heard some nurses talking about Marie Peppers. I was intrigued...something about the way they spoke about her made me realize that this was a lady I needed to meet.

Now, don't get me wrong...I'm always skeptical when things sound a little too good to be true. So I reached out to Marie and grilled her a bit about her programs, wanting to know all the details before going all in.

And then something that happened blew my mind.

You see, I totally expected Marie to try to coax me into buying whatever she was selling. I've heard all these promises before, and I know how the story goes...they always sound tantalizing, but they seem vague. And then you're made to feel like you're missing out by not jumping at the opportunity with both feet (and both eyes closed!).

But that's not at all how Marie reacted. In fact, she did the complete opposite. She sensed my hesitation, and told me plainly that if I don't trust her, I shouldn't sign up for her programs. She had none of that desperate scammer energy that was half begging, half ordering me to just sign up already. She wanted me to do what felt right to me and nothing more.

I can't tell you enough about how Marie has changed my life. That meaning and purpose I'd been searching for, especially since losing Ivy, finally found its way into my life. And of course I'll never get over my loss. Bereavement, especially when it comes to the loss of a child, always stays with you; there is no escaping it. But my angel Ivy knew I needed something to keep going, and she made sure I found it in my life.

So let's talk about numbers, shall we? Because if I was a skeptic, I can accept that you are, too.

More than 4000 nurses have completed Marie's programs, and virtually all of them have secured work from home jobs. And the best part is that this is not just another online program where the person who created it sits at home collecting profits while everyone who purchased it is on his or her own, trying to figure out how to make practical use of all the information. Marie is a nurse in the true sense of the word, in that she's providing service to each and every one of the nurses who joins her programs. She's hands on, goes above and beyond, and will go to the ends of the earth to help her graduates find an amazing work from home job. She even took us on a delightful retreat, where she splurged for all of us to get spa treatments and gourmet food. Marie will go to bat for you in ways you never imagined possible.

I went to end my story on a very personal note. My elderly mother still lives in Zimbabwe, and unfortunately, she's been struggling with congestive heart failure. That alone is a horrible thing to live with here in the land of plenty. But imagine going through it in an African village where there's no clean water in your home. Let's be honest, none of this is Marie's problem, but as always, she was eager to help out. With her help, we were able to drill a well on my mother's property...we named that well Marie Peppers.

I've come a long way from my humble beginnings as the village nanny. And without Marie Peppers, I have no idea where I'd be today. But I get to live out my dream every day, honoring my angel Ivy, all thanks to Marie Peppers. I can't recommend her program more.

Rosemary Matsikidze, LVN

BETTY'S STORY

I didn't know another way. I truly did not.

I'd spent my entire adult life (can you even call an 18 year old an adult??) working in a hospital...the very same hospital, for nearly 40 years.

I'd started out as a phlebotomist while I worked towards my degree in nursing, and over the course of the next 4 decades, I had various jobs in that hospital.

I can't stress this enough...every crack in the wall was familiar to me. Every scratch in the paint; every scuff on the floor. That hospital was my home away from home. And even when my shift ended and I went home, a part of my heart and soul remained in that hospital. You know what I mean...it's a nurse thing.

And the truth is that I was made to be a nurse. I lived, breathed, and slept that job. My patients became my extended family and all of their problems came home with me. I couldn't help it, although I really did try.

But you're a nurse, so you get it. This isn't a job we can wash off at the end of a shift. It's like a second skin we can never take off. And in some ways, that's the beauty of it...we really do care in a way that most other medical professionals don't. But we can't save everyone, no matter how hard we may try. And that becomes a dark cloud hanging over our heads, casting a shadow over everything we do.

In my case, I kept moving higher and higher (up that proverbial totem pole) in various jobs as a nurse at that hospital. I knew I was ridiculously good at what I did. And I was exceptionally proud of that...why wouldn't I be?

Let's be honest here...nursing is unparalleled...you learn on the job, you try your best, sometimes you're just blindly hoping that what you're doing will work, and no one gives you a medal to tell you what a great job you've done. I could go on and on about some of the patients who will forever be etched upon my heart, others who will forever haunt my spirit, and the ones who've run into me in public, raving about what great care I provided them...now half the time, I can't even remember them when I look them in the face! But it's always rewarding, and not for one moment have I ever doubted my decision to become a nurse.

And then one day it all went to hell. Literally.

Ok, maybe not literally. There were no demons, pitchforks, or flames. But it sure felt as if there were.

Our hospital, the one I'd worked (diligently, tirelessly, and rarely even entertaining a single day off!) at since I was a teenager, merged with another local hospital, and I'm pretty sure you can figure out where this is going.

It started out okay, actually. I'd developed a transitional care unit for short-term rehabilitation. I started in that unit as a staff nurse, and ended up as Director of Nursing. And I had an absolutely stellar staff working under me. I was ridiculously (and understandably) proud of that unit. It was a 5 star unit that was renowned in our community. You'd think my position would be secure. But if you did think that, then I'm afraid you thought wrong. And you're not alone because I thought wrong, too.

They shut down the unit because it wasn't a big money maker. It's a sad day when all hospitals can think about is money, as opposed to what everything thinks we're there for...to heal the sick. But that's a whole other story for another day.

Yep, you guessed it...the layoffs began. And the worst part is that it wasn't even the newer employees, or the ones with questionable records. Some of the most outstanding caregivers I've ever seen were sent packing. And many of them had spent their entire careers giving everything they had to the patients at that hospital.

If you figured my turn was coming up, you guessed right again.

I still remember the day vividly, as if it happened yesterday. And it played out like some kind of bad dream, where I desperately wanted to wake up and find myself back at my job...the one I loved before this horrific marriage between two hospitals turned my world upside down.

So there I was walking into that meeting HR called...it felt like I was walking to some kind of witch's hanging...sure enough, I was expected to do something that would have compromised my principles, and before I knew it, I was out of a job. It truly was a witch hunt.

I'm not going to mince words or sugarcoat...I was beyond crushed. The whole experience just broke me. I remember walking out of that hospital, down those halls for the last time, with memories filling up every corner, over the last 4 decades of my life.

I honestly didn't know what to do with myself. Who would hire me now, as an older lady who'd spent the last 40 years being a dutiful nurse for one hospital that readily discarded me like garbage when they determined I was no longer any use to them?

And if I couldn't work as a nurse, what else would I be? I had no other working identity, nor did I want one.

And then life threw a series of hurdles my way that quite literally brought me to my knees. My dad passed away right before I lost my job, so I was already shaken and not exactly walking on steady ground. And then right after I found myself suddenly unemployed, my mother in law unexpectedly died of a stroke. I say "unexpectedly" because she seemed to be in great health, and none of us saw it coming.

But then my real nightmare came along. My 55 year old brother went to work one day with chest pains. He never came home. Not alive, anyway. My brother, who worked so that I could stay home and be a caregiver to our sick mother (what else would I do now that I was no longer employed as a nurse?)...my brother who used to proofread my papers and make them perfect because he insisted I ramble (you be the judge of that since you're reading this, haha), my sweet brother who was a lawyer, but didn't think to leave a will suddenly dropped out of my world.

So what was I supposed to do now? Everyone near and dear to me was dying. My career was over...or was it?

Say what you will, but I truly believe my dear ones who left me to make their way to heaven are angels who put me on the path I'm on now. They led me to my angel on earth...Marie Peppers.

So, where do I even begin with her?

Well, she was working a remote position as a nurse, and it got me wondering about what was possible. She told me she had a program, and here's what's really crazy...I was gifted some money from an unexpected source (talk about angels making all the arrangements for me to pursue this path!), so I used it to enroll in her program.

And then my life completely changed.

With her help, my resume got whittled down to perfection...don't laugh, but it was 6 pages long...somewhere, my brother up in heaven is laughing at how much I rambled.

But there I was, with a crisp, clear, and concise resume, ready to take my first nursing job outside of the toxic environment I'd been forced out of.

And the job offers were (still are!) coming at me from every side. Marie truly is an earth angel because she prepared me for this amazing new career I have...still as a nurse because I wouldn't have it any other way, and still healing humans, but this time, without having to be on my feet all day, without a commute, and without HR asking me to engage in varying degrees of immorality in a hospital where people come because they are literally on the precipice of life and death.

And now, I get to choose the kind of jobs I take, when I want to work, and how I want to make the most use of my nursing degree, years of experience, and all the good stuff that goes along with that.

Here's the thing...I seriously entertained letting my license lapse because what happened to me in that hospital was so traumatizing that I didn't think I could operate as a nurse (other than a caregiver to my mom) ever again.

But with Marie's help, I not only get paid well to be a nurse, I get to do it from home and still care for my mom while I'm at it.

There are signs everywhere. For me, they came in the form of my angels above me connecting me with a rare angel on earth. But if you're reading this, take it as a sign. My angels want you to be happy and fulfilled as a nurse, too. So don't wait another moment to get into Marie's course...your own amazing future is waiting. I promise.

Betty Anderson, RN

JOHN'S STORY

Nursing is like combat. Every day is a battle, lives are on the line, and some days, you feel like your soul is literally being sucked right out of your body through a long, pokey straw.

At times, there's blood everywhere. You often feel like you're dodging bullets. And managers scream instructions in your face, sometimes treating you like a bug they just want to squish and then scrape off the bottom of their shoes.

In case you haven't figured it out yet, I'm a military guy. I did 8 years of active duty, and while you can leave the Navy, the Navy never truly leaves you.

What I mean is...I take a rather no nonsense approach to everything. Just the facts, ma'am, no emotions, just tell it to me straight.

This is not to say that I don't have any emotions. In fact, quite the opposite is true. Emotions are actually the very reason that led me to drop a successful career and become a full-time nurse.

So, here's the deal...my mom got diagnosed with COPD...of all the bombs dropped on my head over the course of my life, this one exploded the loudest, and splattered every part of me across the floor.

After the shock wore off, reality sunk in...my mother was dying.

Someone needed to care for her. And nothing less than the very best would do. I couldn't accept anything else for my mother.

So who best to do that job? Yeah, you guessed it..that would be me. Call me a mama's boy all you want. I'll wear the title proudly. What I needed to do was never in question...I was going to provide my mother the best possible care right up until she earned her wings and moved on to the next plane of existence.

Minor detail...for that, I'd have to become a nurse. No problem. I've been in war zones...nursing school, I can handle.

Well, I could tell you that it was easy, but that would make me a liar. And that I am most certainly not. But my mother was worth everything to me, and there was no schooling on the planet that would have scared me off, no matter how difficult.

So there I was, a 40-something retired military man, a former IT professional (did I mention that that's what I did after leaving the military?) who put away his computer skills, and donned a pair of scrubs, a stethoscope, and some latex gloves. And most of all, I got to be a live-in nurse for my mom until she passed away in 2014 (in case you're wondering, yes, I still miss her).

My first foray into nursing was at a Long Term Care Facility. If you're an LPN, you've probably worked in one of those yourself. Sure, it was different from working on computers, but I caught on, and I turned out to be a really good nurse. I guess my reasons for going into it were so pure that not being great at it didn't seem like an option. The only problem was that after the loss of my mother, I couldn't handle my day job anymore. Too many reminders of my mother, and everything she went through right up until the moment I lost her.

I had to move on to something else for the benefit of my ailing soul. A correctional facility had a job opening, and my military background made me a natural good fit for it. What I didn't realize at the time was that this sort of work was considered some of the most challenging in the field of nursing. Not knowing that was probably a blessing, though, because I didn't see it as terribly difficult. All I knew was that I needed to keep helping people without getting too emotionally attached.

I was an agency nurse...in case you don't know what that means, it's one of those nurses who picks up a new contract for two to six months at a time, which, of course, made it much easier not to get attached, since I never stayed around any of my patients for very long. The downside was that just every facility has its own rules and procedures, and they're not big on spending much time teaching any of those things to new contract nurses. With barely any orientation, I was expected to hit the ground running and make myself useful, even though I was basically always that new kid in class whom everyone stares at, and who's trying to remember where the bathroom is located.

It hit me one day that I just wasn't happy. And it wasn't just the constantly changing environment, either.

Let's be honest here...you're a nurse, so you know the downsides of nursing...the environments we work in are often toxic, and playing politics is sometimes more important than actual patient care. For me, personally (and maybe this is because of what happened to my mother, but I suspect this is true of many nurses), I struggled to dissociate myself at the end of each shift. Taking my patients' pain home with me was a sort of demented takeout that weighed down on my shoulders (and my spirit) every day, and there was no receptacle I could just toss it into...I was stuck with it. Some part of me was ready to walk away from nursing, but the rest of me just couldn't do it. By this time, nursing coursed through my veins, and nothing in the world could ever take its place in my life.

But how could I reconcile that with all the struggles I was having?

Remote nursing came upon my radar, but it was something of an urban legend, in that every nurse had "heard" about it, but no one actually knew someone who was doing it.

And let's not kid ourselves...remote nursing is the holy grail of nursing. Every nurse dreams about it, but was it even a real thing? I mean, did such a thing truly exist, or was this like those UFO sightings that many people have allegedly had, but no one seems to have any actual evidence of alien existence.

What I didn't realize at the time was that my life was about to change.

Now, when I think back on my life as a nurse, there have been two pivotal moments. One was the reason I dropped my (then) existing career in order to become a nurse.

And the other was when I met Marie Peppers.

The first one was bad, even though it ultimately led to something good because I absolutely LOVE being a nurse.

The second one was so amazing, I can't even quite find the words to describe it.

So let's talk a bit about Marie Peppers....

I found her on Facebook, joined her group, and just sort of lurked for a bit. I mean, I'm a skeptic, and I've heard of all the promises so many snake oil salesmen out there make...give me your money and I'll hand over the goods.

I'm not one to part with my money easily, not so much because of the cash itself, but rather, it's the principle of it. I'm not going to be swindled into making some charlatan rich.

But Marie Peppers restored my faith in humanity. Not only is her program amazing, but even when I was done with it, she wasn't done with me. Not till I had a job I loved (and am still happily doing every Monday through Friday!).

You see, I finished her program, applied to jobs, but at first, the rejections were coming at me from every side. I wasn't too shaken. I mean, that sort of thing happens in every industry, right?

But Marie knew better, mainly because she's put together a program that, if you do all the things, you absolutely WILL land an amazing remote nursing job.

It didn't take long for Marie to figure out where I was making mistakes both in my resume AND in my interviews. And after that, it was literally like magic…I had not one but TWO job offers! And they both offered amazing benefits, great pay, and the best job site on the planet…my living room!

Marie Peppers is my miracle. Literally. She made it possible for me to continue working as a nurse, to enjoy working as a nurse, and most of all, to put the skills I've learned as a nurse to use to save lives without spending my days in a toxic environment.

And you know the running joke with nurses is that we'll work till we're dead, and *maybe* we'll only work a partial shift on the day of our funeral. But here's what's even crazier…I don't *want* to stop doing this remote nursing job because it pays well, gives me every holiday and weekend off (yes, you read that right…can you believe there's *any* nursing job that does that??), and it doesn't wear down my body (12-16 hour shifts, anyone?) or my soul. I get to help people while living my best life *ever*.

If I can do this, you can, too. Being a nurse does *not* require you to be a martyr, I promise. Connect with Marie Peppers, so that you can have your dream job as a nurse. And so that you can sleep in on Saturdays because I always do, and so can you, my friend. Just go for it…you've got everything to gain, and nothing in the world to lose.

John Tygart, LVN

VICTORIA'S STORY

So, yeah, I'm one of those...my mom was a nurse; my dad was a doctor...of course I became a nurse. What else would I be?

But for me, there was more to it than that.

See, my dad, the doctor...the one who healed others, who made disease go away (that's how I saw him, anyway), who turned sickness into health...was diagnosed with cancer when I was a teenager. And the one thing my dad couldn't cure was himself.

I watched him deteriorate before my eyes. It wasn't long before he couldn't work and support us anymore, so my mom went back to full time nursing...night shift. And guess who was left in charge?

Make no mistake; I didn't resent it one bit. I was actually happy that I could care for my ailing daddy. And I don't just mean fluffing his pillow and getting him some hot tea, either. When he needed someone to clean him up after yet another bout of vomiting, I was there. I changed his sheets, and cleaned him up as his cancer progressed. At some point, my dad started to lose control of his bowels, and with Mom at work, I was the one who took care of everything he needed. So there was no question about what I wanted to do once I grew up...my dad's cancer (and death...he died right after I finished high school) forced me to grow up a bit early. And I was already a nurse...before I'd even set foot into a single classroom where the basics of nursing were taught.

Now, here's the thing...I was the oldest of 4 kids, and that may

MARIA BRUSCINI-PEPPERS, LPN

have been fine on a doctor's salary. But once Dad was gone, money was tight, and my mom had become a single mother, trying her best to raise all of us on a nurse's salary.

What I'm trying to say is that there was no money for me to go to college. I had to put myself through school, which didn't exactly put me in a class of my own. But it certainly added a layer of complication to my life. I dropped out and took a gap year, working as a bank teller in order to help my mom with money, so that she and my siblings could grieve. What I didn't realize (but believe me, it caught up to me later) was that I never got a chance to truly grieve.

At some point, I made my way back to school...life has to go on, doesn't it? I went about this old school...at a simple, old-fashioned hospital-based program, where I went to class in the morning, worked as a phlebotomist at the hospital in the afternoons and evenings, and worked night shifts (like mother, like daughter, right?) on Fridays and Saturdays at the emergency department. Sound exhausting? Trust me, it was!

But I still graduated at the top of my class and went straight to work in a trauma ICU at a Philadelphia hospital.

Yeah, it sounds impressive. But remember how I mentioned that I never really got to grieve my father's early demise at the hands of cancer?

Well, if you've never worked in an ICU, let me tell you something... every patient seems to be somewhere in between living and dying, and emotions are understandably running high. With the patients, with their families, and even with us because if you're a nurse reading this, you know how much each patient means to us, even if they were only in our care for a short time. I couldn't help thinking about my father, and how unfair it seemed that he lost his battle after helping so many others win theirs. And it's not that I'd begrudge any of my dad's former patients. It's that being in the ICU and seeing people so desperately clinging to the vestiges of life left me feeling vulnerable and fragile. It had a way of bringing back everything that happened to my dad. Except here I was, an adult now, caring for strangers who (together with their families) were relying on me to get them back on their feet (or at least out of the ICU!).

But I'd seen this play out before when I was a teenager, and it seemed to be like Groundhog Day on a repeat loop, showing up in my life over and over again, like a cruel reminder of the loss I'd already suffered, but never got a chance to properly grieve.

Now don't get me wrong...I have so many fond memories of patients I took care of in the ICU. And if circumstances had been different, maybe I'd even still be there because you know what they say about patterns in our life repeating themselves, right?

Well, I didn't really get a say in the matter. And it's funny how life sometimes chooses our path for us, isn't it?

Let me explain....

So, in my case, cliche as it may sound, I was always sick and tired. Literally. It seemingly came out of nowhere, but I felt crappy, and I could have slept all day and all night, and still felt exhausted. And if you haven't worked in the ICU, I'm sure you can still imagine how exhausting that could be for anyone...much less for someone whose default state has suddenly become "sick and tired."

At first, I did what all nurses tend to do...I ignored it and kept going. I had patients who needed me, and I reasoned that they were sicker and probably more tired than I was. But this wasn't going away on its own.

Everything came to a head on Labor Day of 2003 (can you believe that was nearly 20 years ago already??). There I was with my husband and two young kids at our little condo on the shore, trying hard to enjoy a holiday weekend.

But I couldn't.

My stomach hurt so much that I couldn't even think about eating. I was so bloated that my husband's sweatpants were all that (barely) fit me. And on a scale of 1-10, the pain I was in was at least a 12. I knew I was in trouble…I had ovarian cancer; I was certain of it. As a nurse, I'd seen this before. I knew the symptoms. I was absolutely convinced that I was dying.

So I did what any nurse (who's also a wife and mother) would do… I gritted my teeth and bore through the pain, hopped in my car, and drove home in Labor Day traffic, leaving my hubby and kiddos wondering what the heck just happened. And I checked myself into the local ER (but not before first paying the mortgage for the month because poor Hubby had no idea how), bracing myself for the horrific diagnosis I just knew was coming.

I still remember the tests, the doctor looking at me with a mixture of concern and pity, and the deep breath he took before opening his mouth to tell me that I had ~~ovarian cancer~~ Crohn's disease. The doctor looked stern as he told me it was a chronic illness, there was no cure, and I would need to take immune suppressing medication the rest of my life. He expected me to be despondent.

I was overjoyed, and could have kissed him…I wasn't dying! I felt like I'd gotten another chance at life.

But I quickly realized that working as a floor nurse in an ICU just wasn't an option anymore. I could tell you all about the different things I tried…working in an assisted living facility, working as a medicare wellness nurse…God knows I tried every which way to remain a nurse. But Crohn's disease seemed to win the battle every single time. And all my waking hours were spent working, anyway. I'd come home way too wiped out to do simple tasks like putting my kids to bed.

I tried to retire; I really did. I was willing to let Crohn's have the last word. My kids were older; they didn't need me for everything anymore…maybe it was time to just relax and accept my illness as having a final say over everything I do.

But if you're a nurse, you know it's easier said than done. I am certain that among all the blood types...A, O, B, AB, there's another one that no one speaks of...NURSE. Let's be honest...nursing is in our blood. We can't not be nurses. It's like its own sort of torture, just sitting around and not using our hands to heal. I needed to do something more than relaxing and enjoy retirement.

That's when I learned about Marie Peppers.

Now let me backtrack a tiny bit...I can divide my working life into three categories...each of them representing a major event that shaped the trajectory of my career.

The first was my father dying, and the care I put into making the final months of his life as comfortable a possible.

The second was finding out I have an incurable disease that required a bare minimum of 12 hours of sleep...in a career where 12 hour shifts (and they're never JUST 12 hours, are they?) are the norm.

The third was finding Marie Peppers' program that allowed me to continue being a nurse without having to leave my house.

Honestly, I never wanted to retire, and I certainly didn't want this disease to win. But to continue being a nurse, I had to find a different way, and that's EXACTLY what Marie brought into my life.

I took her program, got a job offer almost immediately, and by year 2 of working from home, I got a raise AND a promotion. And the best part...I get to continue to take care of other people's health without compromising my own.

I can't even begin to tell you just how much Marie Peppers changed my life. And I know she can do the same to yours. You don't have to have a chronic illness to want to work from home, especially with a modern day plague that shows no signs of slowing down all around us.You don't have to require 12 hours of sleep or simply not feel like you want to spend 12 hours (or more!) on your feet every day. And most of all, you don't have to work in some medical facility and play politics all day in order to make a difference in people's lives as a nurse.

One thing I can tell you for sure is that you've earned this…a good life, an ideal work/life balance, and a job that pays you well without sucking the life out of you. Sign up for Marie's program… I promise it'll be one of the best decisions you'll ever make!

Victoria Knotts, BSN, RN-BC

NICOLE'S STORY

My career in nursing started out on Wall Street.

Ok, well, not exactly. But that's where the shift happened...that knowledge that I was in the wrong place, and I needed to find another career path.

Now, if I'm honest (and we're all friends here, right?), I'd have to admit that my career in nursing started...and abruptly ended, when I entered nursing school at 18 (don't judge me; I was still a teenager) and flunked out because I didn't put enough effort into it. I mean, nursing is a fairly common career choice (but we still have this crazy shortage of nurses!), so I figured getting through my education would be a breeze.

It wasn't. At all.

So there I was, a single mom, working as a collector on Wall Street.

And while it sounds glamorous (I mean, it's Wall Street), I was struggling with money, and the realization that I couldn't keep this up...it wasn't fair to my son...for much longer. I needed to try nursing again...it called to me.

And this time, at 27, I had matured, and had been around the block a lot more times than when I was 18. I went into it prepared.

Here's what was different...this time, I was a single mom...with a full time job. At 18, I was unencumbered, and could have focused just on my classes. Now I had a child who depended on me, a job

I had to go to in order to keep a roof over our heads, and nursing classes (remember, on a subject that I'd flunked out before, under much easier circumstances) on top of it all.

But the stakes were higher, so I had no excuses. I got my ASN, passed my NCLEX, and packed up myself and my son, and made the move from New York to Florida.

Next thing I knew, I was a bedside nurse in South Florida, working in a Progressive Care Unit. I was doing what I loved every day, and I knew that I'd earned it. Completely high on nursing, I decided to go for my BSN and then my MSN...may as well go for the gusto, right? I was determined to invest in myself to have the greatest possible opportunities as a nurse.

And then I started passing out at work.

No, I don't mean merely feeling faint, or tired, or overworked, or exhausted, or dealing with a bit of vertigo.

I was out cold on the floor of the hospital, and not just once or twice. This became routine.

Now, let's not kid ourselves...you don't have to be a nurse to know that this isn't normal.

And then more symptoms came on, as if there were some kind of hellish party going on in my body.

First came the horrific headaches...the kind that make you think your head is going to explode and fly off into another dimension. Then the chest pains, which were quickly joined by tachycardia. My blood pressure was always either too high or too low. I could tell you that I might have ignored the fainting, but that would have been insane because that alone was really serious. But tack this bevy of symptoms on, and I had no choice but to seek medical help.

POTS. That's the diagnosis I was given.

Postural Orthostatic Tachycardia Syndrome. It's a form of dysautonomia.

If you've not run into it as a nurse, let me give you the Cliffs Notes version…basically, it affects the autonomic nervous system, which regulates bodily functions we don't consciously control (or even think about!), like heart rate, blood pressure, sweating, and body temperature…just to name a few.

And if that weren't enough, there's a lower amount of blood being circulated, excessive pooling of blood below the heart when upright, and elevated levels of certain hormones, like epinephrine, for instance.

So, yeah, my body was a mess.

And the best part? It seems POTS is brought on by stress, fatigue, and standing too long (hello, bedside nurse life!).

And while POTS can be controlled, there is no cure.

Everything I worked for was essentially being taken from me. I had to leave bedside nursing…what choice did I have? It's kind of like learning that you have a peanut allergy, when your favorite food is peanut butter pie…you don't *want* to give up that thing you love, but if you don't, it will kill you. Literally.

Luckily, I didn't have to leave nursing altogether. I was able to secure a non-clinical position in the same facility, as a Cardiac Nurse Navigator. My job was to follow cardiac patients from admission to discharge, and beyond. This program was designed to decrease readmission, which is especially dangerous for cardiac patients. It was actually quite rewarding and enjoyable, plus I went from 12-15 hour shifts, to 8 hour shifts. And I wasn't expected to be on my feet the whole time.

Still, POTS made every day a struggle in my new position, but luckily, I had more good days than bad.

Just as everything seemed to be falling into place, the pandemic came along, and tore our world apart.

And everything changed. I was forced to leave my (non-essential!) position and work as a bedside nurse in a COVID unit. But how could I do that? My disease made the demands of a job like that impossible to fulfill. And contracting COVID with POTS would have been catastrophic for me.

Once again, I was at a crossroads, and needed to pivot to something different. But I'd worked too hard, and come too far (remember, I got my BSN and MSN) to give up on nursing. This was my career for life.

They say that every storm leaves a rainbow in its wake. And Marie Peppers came into my life like the much-needed rainbow I was desperately seeking. I decided to once again invest in myself and my career by enrolling in her program.

And what a difference it's made!

I still get to work as a nurse, but from the comfort of my home.

If I'm having a bad day (thanks, POTS!), I can still work from home, and don't have to call in sick, like I had to, back when I worked in a medical facility.

No more standing for long periods of time, no more commute, no more of the chaos that's just par for the course when you're a nurse in a hospital.

Here's what I want to tell you…there are SO many ways to be a nurse. And you don't have to be a bedside nurse on your feet all day to make a difference in people's lives. You don't have to leave the comfort of your sofa to be effective as a nurse. You can be a healer at home, without having to go anywhere.

I honestly don't know what I'd have done if I hadn't found Marie and her amazing course.

But what I do know with 100% certainty is that Marie made it possible for me to continue my lifelong dream of making a meaningful difference in people's lives (not to mention making a very solid living!) as a nurse. I couldn't be more grateful!

Nicole Felix, MSN, RN

MELISSA'S STORY

So, you may want to brace yourselves because my story is a bit rough around the edges...but all's well that ends well, right?

Well, I'm a country gal, a Georgia peach, if you will. And I was raised in a lovely, rural part of Georgia by parents who worked day and night to keep a roof over our heads, and food on the table for me, my younger sister, and my baby brother. We didn't have much, at least not as far as material things went. But we had enough love to fill an ocean, plus a whole lot of faith. Sundays were spent at church in the morning, and then at Grandma's for lunch in the afternoon. I have enough memories to fill a bottomless box, of spending those days with all my aunts and uncles and cousins, running around Grandma's yard. Like I said, we didn't have a lot of stuff. But God made sure I was always surrounded by people who loved me.

Watching my parents work themselves to exhaustion certainly influenced me. I had a dream...don't we all when we're in that idealistic stage of childhood?

My sister and I made a pact of sorts...she'd become a doctor, and I'd become a nurse, and between the two of us, we'd make enough money to buy enormous mansions, side by side (of course...it starts with sharing a room, and soon you're sharing a huge plot of land), with a house for Mom and Dad in the back.

It didn't exactly happen that way.

I went into the army right out of high school, just as my daddy had before me. I was shipped off to Germany, where I lived for a while. I was there to watch the Berlin Wall fall, and to this day, I love that I got to witness such a significant moment in history. It's a story I share with my 4 children, and they've shared it as well.

Well, somewhere along the way, the road to my childhood dreams became bumpy and winding.

While I was still in the army, I got married, had a baby, came home, and soon found myself divorced. And there I was, a single mother to the most beautiful baby girl on the planet (I mean, you could debate me on that, but you'd lose). I had all the love in the world for her. But that's pretty much all I had.

So I had no choice but to move back with my parents. It wasn't ideal, but I was grateful that it was even an option. I took a job in a sewing mill to provide for my little family. And then I met my second husband. And became pregnant with another perfect little girl. And then my second husband left me.

So now I had two little girls to raise on my own. There was only so much burden I could place on my parents (remember, they barely made ends meet with their own children), so I applied for and received low income housing, and took a job in a cotton mill...the same one my parents worked in. It gave a whole new perspective to the concept of "we're all family here" in the workplace.

And then my world was turned upside down. My teenage brother was diagnosed with an extremely aggressive form of colon cancer. Exactly 6 months later, he earned his wings. My family was shattered in ways I can't even begin to put into words. Speaking strictly for myself, my faith was lost. Where was God? Why didn't He let my little brother grow up?

It's weird how fate works. On the night my brother died, I met husband number 3. Yep, you guessed it, I got pregnant soon afterward. And he left me. I was a single mom...again...to a growing brood. My future as a nurse seemed farther and farther away. My husband and I attempted to reconcile...and I became pregnant with baby number 4. My blessings kept on multiplying. I'll never see my children as burdens...they're absolute blessings. But my dreams seemed to be on the other side of the world...and totally unreachable.

I could fill you in on all the details of working in that cotton mill for 15 years. But let's skip to the good part.

They say life begins at 40, right? Well, for me, that may be especially apt because I started nursing school at the tender age of 40.

Soon enough, I'd earned my LPN, and my sister started school to become a PA...not *quite* a doctor, but close enough. So we did both fulfill our dreams and we carried out that pact, even if it didn't happen the easy, fast, and romantic way we'd envisioned it as children.

Were all my struggles behind me at that point? Not quite.

My grandson died at 5 months of age, at the hands of a negligent babysitter. I remember sitting vigil at his side, along with my children and their spouses, surrounding my grandbaby with love, just as my parents and extended family did with me when I was a little girl. We donated his organs, saving 4 different babies' lives in the process. As tragic as my grandson's death was, I take comfort in knowing that he gave the gift of life. And it also taught me a valuable lesson as a healer...a life, no matter how short, is still a lifetime.

I've been a nurse for a decade now. But, oh, how I crammed so many years into that decade. I have worked in LTC, Med-Surg, Trauma, Hospice, and Home Health. Over the last 4 years, I've worked as a private duty pediatric nurse for respiratory children with trachs, vents, etc. Has it been easy? Absolutely not! But I finally clawed my way out of the financial struggle that I was born into. And I was able to provide for my children...and I'm spoiling the daylights out of my grandchildren...and they've made every difficult shift worthwhile.

Here's what nobody tells you about nursing while you're still dreaming about doing it...it's only been 10 years, and granted, I was well-seasoned by the time I became a nurse, but my body is downright *ravaged*. Bedside nursing is rewarding beyond description, but boy, does it ever take its toll. My knees, my hips, my back, my shoulders...everything hurts. Literally.

Now, did you think this was going to make me give up nursing? Bless your heart! I did NOT come this far, work this hard, and get through all those crappy things to just give up.

But I also knew I had to find another way. Humans just weren't built to do bedside nursing for the entire span of their career.

And that's when I learned about Marie Peppers, and her amazing courses.
Not gonna lie...I was hesitant. I mean, could this one course *really* help me get a job as a remote nurse? Surely, it had to be more complicated than that, right? What was the catch...?

I stalked her group for over a year before taking the plunge. My only regret is not going for it sooner.

It just took a few short months to finish her course, and 3 weeks after that, I had my first interview. I ended up getting a job as a Chronic Care Manager, and I've never looked back.

Of all the jobs I've taken as a nurse, and I've listed them above, so you can see that there have been A LOT, this has, by far and away, been the most rewarding job I've done as a nurse. Nothing makes me happier than building relationships with patients, and guiding them to make better healthcare decisions.

But it gets better from there...I've recently been promoted into management...to recruit, hire, and train nurses to do what I do now...and this job has a great salary, full benefits, and bonuses! Y'all, pinch me!

I'd never be here without Marie Peppers. I'm certain she was sent to me by my angels...my baby brother, and my baby grandson. And I couldn't be more grateful.

Don't wait for angels to push Marie into your life. Take my word for it...this is the best career decision you'll ever make...don't put it off another moment!

Melissa English, LPN

JESSICA'S STORY

My story isn't like most, so you may want to grab a chair for this one.

Ok, deep breath, so...my childhood dream wasn't to become a nurse. At all.

I wanted to be a teacher. And who knows, maybe every little girl goes through a stage where she wants to be a teacher.

But I showed signs of being a healer since I was a toddler. I don't remember any of this, but my mom says that I was eager to help take care of my grandpa when he was at the end of his life...as a toddler, mind you.

Not to mention, I was *that* kid...who stuck up for the bullied kids, who helped the elderly get their mail, who pleaded with my parents to stop the car when there was a dead animal on the side of the road...so I could take it home and bury it.

So maybe I didn't want to be a nurse, but somehow, nursing wanted me.

If only it were that simple. I mean...if only we had the wisdom we have now, in hindsight, when we were young and making all these decisions.

One thing I'll say for me, I was a good student. So as I approached college, my options were pretty unlimited. I did initially choose nursing, but for all the wrong reasons...I had this idea in my head that nurses make A LOT of money. And teachers...well, you know what they say about teachers taking second jobs just to get by.

But I didn't end up going to college for nursing after all, nor did I become a teacher.

You know how life has an uncanny ability to get in the way, and effectively make decisions for us?

Well, guess what...I became a wife, and then a mom, and that (rightfully) became my number one focus. So I opted to work nights, while my husband worked days, so that we could avoid (ridiculously high) childcare expenses. I spent the next ten years waitressing at an Irish pub.

Sure, it was a far cry from nursing, but in an odd, roundabout way, waitressing prepared me for the rigors of being a nurse. Of course, at the time, I had no idea I'd end up a nurse. I was just living in the moment. I made good money, great friends, and a suitable mommy life for my kiddos.

Maybe you're wondering how I survived taking care of children by day, while working all night. Nah, if you've ever been a clinical nurse in a hospital, you already know what that's like. So let's not waste time on those details.

But ultimately, I knew I couldn't be a waitress forever, and as my children reached a certain age, I had a whole new set of decisions to make.

So, the year was 2007 (seems like just yesterday, but can you believe how long ago it was??), and I was making another attempt at becoming a nurse. This time I was older, wiser, with more life experience, and perhaps going after a career in nursing for the right reasons...not for the money, which, while good, will never (on its own) make nursing worth it. There was a two year ASN program I wanted to get into, and it was actually quite competitive, but I managed to get in! I can't even begin to tell you how excited I was.

What I underestimated was how difficult being an "older student" would be, and I'm not going to lie...there were days I didn't think I'd find my way to the finish line. On many a morning, my son would make me coffee before leaving for school because he'd find me asleep over a textbook.

But there I was in 2011, graduating, while my husband and children cheered me on.

My first post-graduation job was at a facility for people with developmental disabilities. The place was beyond gorgeous and glossy, like the 5 star hotel version of a medical facility. The work was a lot less glamorous, but seeing how happy we made the patients made me happy. And that made every day worthwhile.

Fast forward to 2016...my husband got an offer to relocate through his company to South Carolina...the thought of a warmer climate definitely appealed to me. Our children were grown by then, and moving out on their own. So off we went.

My first job in a new state was working as a private duty nurse with trach/vent babies in their homes. Babies were new to me (other than the ones I raised, of course), and yeah, I did have a momentary panic of "you're not leaving your fragile child in *my* hands, are you?" But I absolutely loved the work; it was SO rewarding! And then my duties expanded to traveling statewide to do supervisor visits and admissions.

As I look back, this is where my burnout began. There were just so many patients in need, but not enough staff. The hours were long; the travel was constant. And there were enough charts to paper every wall in my house. I knew it was time for a change.

I ended up getting hired to work at a brand new geri/psych unit at the local hospital. I was hired for the night shift (my waitressing days beckoned, sort of like the ghost of Christmas past) three nights a week, PLUS two 10 hour day shifts doing private duty with one family who had a sick toddler. Just writing this makes me feel tired…and I can't imagine reading it doesn't make you feel the same way. It was madness, and looking back, maybe I do have a bit of bionic woman in me. I honestly think ALL nurses do.

And then…a miracle happened. I met Marie Peppers. A year of this insanity (3 nights, 2 days of nursing a week) went by before Marie and I met, but maybe that's what I needed to jump on the opportunity Marie placed before me.

Now, at first, we were coworkers…she joined the unit at our hospital.

But Marie was in the process of writing her CCM course, and I was naturally curious…I never dreamed that I'd be able to get a remote job as a nurse.

And then COVID came around, and changed everyone's reality. But for nurses, this had an entirely different meaning. We were essential workers…mandated to work in the COVID units, with zero training, and we were painfully short staffed.
You know when you ask the Universe to give you a sign? Or maybe you don't, but you get a sign that you can't ignore?

Well, I didn't need further motivation. I finished Marie's course before the end of 2020, and with Marie's help, I had three job offers that first week!

I've now been working from home for over a year, and couldn't be happier. In fact, I've even taken a part-time position in Marie's program, assisting students and prospective students.

How has my life changed? Ok, do you have all day…? Let me count the ways….

I have dinner with my family every night. My dogs are well-exercised because running around with them every day is part of my routine. No more crazy commute, no more spending money on lunches, no more running around on my feet all day (other than with my dogs, of course).

And I owe all of this to Marie. I wish I could find the words to express how grateful I am, but sadly, I'm not a poet. All I can tell you is that there absolutely *is* another way to be a nurse, with all of the rewards, and none of the downsides. So go for it. One thing I can absolutely guarantee is that you'll look back on this as one of the greatest decisions you've ever made!

Jessica Christopher, RN

TINA'S STORY

For me, it was a no brainer.

I mean, nursing literally was my professional life.

Let me back up a bit, and fill you in on my backstory.

So, the year was 2019, and I'm still not sure how we're even living in the 20s now...time seems to be flying by, but I digress.

I was 58, so not exactly old, but not a spring chicken, either. I couldn't even begin to fathom a new profession, but let me explain why that was even a teeny tiny thought in my head.

So...I've been a nurse since 1994. Prior to that, I worked in long term facilities in other capacities...as a patient care coordinator, social services...all roads led to nursing. So I got my LPN, and got right down to business...I absolutely loved (still love!) being a nurse. Caring for others always drew me in...the only "work" I've done in my life that wasn't in a medical setting was being a fulltime mother...which is a whole other level of caring for others, but again, I digress.

Now, here's the thing...I'm an anomaly (that means an exception, unusual, a weirdo) among nurses, in that I've only worked three different jobs in my entire 25 year (remember, this was back in 2019) span as a nurse. Most nurses have worked in many different jobs, at many different capacities, in many different facilities. I don't know if I was lucky (since I had stability from staying so long at any given job), or not (since starting a new job, and even looking for one, applying to one, interviewing, you get the idea, was not something I was used to), but there I was, staring down the end of my nursing career...potentially.

Let me explain....

I worked for a nurse practitioner in her clinic, and there were only three humans working there...me, her, and a phlebotomist. It was a clinic that provides bioidentical hormone therapy. I loved my job; that wasn't the issue.

So, what was the issue, you ask?

Well, remember, without the nurse practitioner running the show, there was no show for me to show up to. When the nurse practitioner announced that she planned on retiring and effectively closing up shop in 2021, I knew I'd have to find another job.

Now, if you're reading this, you're a nurse, so I don't have to tell you how physically taxing nursing is, and how it's hard enough at 28, but at 58, you might mistake your daily job for being in hell... literally. And all I could see myself doing, as far as available jobs that I qualified for were concerned, required 12 hour shifts at a long-term facility. In other words, welcome to hell.

Now, remember what I said before, I LOVE nursing. Loved it then, still love it now...I have no plans to slow down or stop.

BUT...being on my feet 12 hours a day just didn't sound good, or even doable. I needed another plan.

I prayed about it, asking God to send me a sign, a clue, a suggestion...something.

What God delivered was SO much better than that...and way beyond my wildest expectations.

So, I found out about an online program I could take, in order to qualify for work from home nursing opportunities. And let's be honest...what nurse wouldn't want to do her job from the comfort of her sofa??

And that's how Marie Peppers came into my life...she was the one who created the program...and talk about under promising and over delivering....

Now, here's the thing...while the nurse practitioner at my prior job had clear plans to retire, we were still open for business, and I had no plans to abandon her. The great thing was that I was able to take one work from home job AND continue to work for that nurse practitioner...it was a thing of beauty, and a dream come true, really. My boss (the nurse practitioner) supported my goals 100%.

And then 2020 rolled around, and Covid became a part of our world.

So, remember how I told you that our clinic provided bioidentical hormones? Well, the thing about that is that it deemed us non-essential (although I'm certain some menopausal women would beg to differ!), and we had to shut down.

Don't get me wrong, we'd have loved to keep going. But my boss was taking care of her mother, who was in hospice. The risk of her getting infected and then passing that on to her mother was too great, and the consequences, too dire. And, of course, we idealistically (or was it foolishly??) believed that Covid would come and go within a few months. As you know, it didn't exactly happen that way.

Now, more than ever, I needed to work from home.

Let me tell you something...before I even go into all the details of how fabulous my life is, now that I don't have to commute, be on my feet all day, play politics in a hospital...I could go on and on... trust me on that.

But, as they say in infomercials, wait...there's more!

Marie's program is not just about learning the requisite information to be a work from home nurse. No...it's SO much more.

For starters, Marie helped me spruce up my resume...I got a call almost immediately upon sending it out.

Then she helped me tweak my interviewing skills...on a zoom call.

Did Marie have to do those things? Absolutely not. All she promised was the program I signed up and paid for.

But remember what I said earlier about under promising and over delivering?

Well, with Marie's help, my resume got me an interview promptly, and I had a job offer less than a week later...I wasn't sure what shocked me more...how quickly I got an amazing job, or how much MONEY they were going to pay me to do it. It was definitely one of those "excuse me while I pick my jaw up off the floor" moments.

Do you want to know what my days look like now?

I start my morning with some coffee and devotions. And then I take calls throughout the day from my sofa, with my Yorkie as my assistant, keeping me company while I work. And on my breaks (lunch, etc), I relax in my backyard, again, with my Yorkie by my side...can you even imagine that kind of life, especially if YOUR days are spent doing 12 hour shifts on your feet that make you feel like you've just run across town, being chased by zombies, all the while knowing that you get to do it all over again the next day?

I asked God for a sign and he sent me an angel...God is another one who over delivers, and I couldn't be more grateful for that.

If you're sitting on the fence, let me do you a favor and push you off. Sign up for Marie's program...you'll start to feel like some part of your life began once you've met Marie...trust me, if you take her program and consort with her, you'll know EXACTLY what I'm talking about...do it!

Tina Houston, LPN

LISA'S STORY

Hmmmmm, where do I even begin...well, let me start by saying that my story is not the typical story you usually hear about nurses. It's not a rags to riches story (or rather, the nurse version of that story), and what I mean by that is that I wasn't a single mother desperate for a solid income...that's not why I became a nurse.

On the contrary, my husband holds a very high position at a company, and my salary isn't even needed.

But I think that this is what makes my story interesting...I chose to be a nurse. I LOVE being a nurse. I have the heart and soul of a nurse. Being a nurse is a tremendous part of my identity.

Nursing is in my blood and DNA. Literally. My mother is a nurse, and she's the one with the typical story of raising me as a single mom and needing a rock solid career that paid well enough for her to take care of me all by herself.

But before I go any deeper into my story, let me introduce myself and tell you a few things about me....

My name is Lisa Brooks, and here's what you need to know about me:

1. I'm a mom to the two most amazing children on the planet...and sure, maybe I'm *a little bit* biased, but I'm sticking to that as an absolute fact.

2. I live with a chronic illness, specifically, fibromyalgia. I don't know if you know too much about it, but it has a way of making you pretty miserable. I won't bore you with the details, but think constant pain, perpetual exhaustion (no matter how many hours of sleep I get), and hot flashes (who knew those had a place outside of menopause, right?).
3. Fibromyalgia is something that makes being a nurse a million times harder, but I did and do manage. And I will continue to.
4. Did I mention how much I absolutely love being a nurse?!

So, here's the thing...I worked as a PACU nurse, and if you're a nurse, I can't imagine you need me to go too deeply into explaining what that's like. But let me just skim the surface a bit...so...as you know, PACU nurses are highly skilled...we take over patient care after surgery. Yeah, it pays well. And yeah, it's exhausting even if you're a fresh out of nursing school 22 year old who barely tips the scale at 100 pounds, and wouldn't know a hot flash from rug burn.

Now, here's the other thing...I get it...surgery is serious business, and it's a lot for any human to process. But let's just say that more often than not, PACU patients don't come out of surgery like a ray of sunshine. The job is rewarding, but also challenging, and there were many days when I smiled through a good bit of frustration.

But I digress....

You see, I wanted to go PRN and work two days a week just because fibromyalgia was making my days harder and harder to get through, even with the smiliest patients on the planet.

But then Covid hit, and everything went to hell. Literally.

And no, it's not even because I was afraid of getting sick and then bringing it home to my two young children.

It was the PPE that made my hot flashes look like child's play by comparison...I was so hot that sweat was pouring off me, which isn't a good look when you're taking care of someone with a fresh surgical wound in the middle of a modern day plague.

It was nurses retiring left and right, and just walking off the job because every day had a way of killing your soul just a little bit more.

It was patients needing so much more care and attention because Covid meant no visitors. Simple tasks that visiting family members used to do, like hand them their drink off their tray table were suddenly a constant duty of mine. Not to mention helping them through their feelings of loneliness and isolation. Because let's face it, being in a surgical center (as a patient) is no one's fantasy. Imagine having to do it all by yourself, with no one who loves you by your side.

And it was my children being out of school and doing remote learning...someone had to be home to supervise them, and my husband wasn't about to leave his top of the corporate ladder job to do it, not that I'd expect him to.

Now, hear me out...I was not just a good nurse (and employee), I was a GREAT one. And again, maybe I'm biased, but I showed up for my patients every single day, no matter how crappy fibromyalgia made me feel, and I went way above and beyond for them. I truly was born to be a healer, and I didn't become a nurse to do the bare minimum.

So I asked my boss once again to let me go PRN. I mean, someone had to be home with my kids, and surely this time around, he'd understand? We were all reeling from the pandemic, everyone was stressed, antsy, and overworked, so how could anyone fault me for having to show up as a mom, especially because, unlike many of the other nurses, I wasn't eager to just walk off the job.

Yep, you guessed it...I got another resounding NO as an answer. So finally, I did walk off the job because what else could I do?

But remember what I said before, being a nurse is in my DNA (I get it from my mama). I don't know how to not be a nurse, and frankly, I don't want to know. Saying goodbye to being a nurse would be like a part of my soul dying. And I value my soul too much to let that happen.

Call it theatrical, overdramatic, or whatever you want to call it, but it's fair to say that Marie Peppers saved my soul. Not because she's Jesus in the flesh (but if you work with her, it may feel that way sometimes, I promise). But rather, because she provided me with a way to continue being a nurse that was in line with the schedule my kids needed (remember, mom duty), that allowed me to work the hours that suit me, that allowed me to work with NO PPE (and I sometimes work in my jammies, so I managed to kick that up a notch or two), and get this...it allows me to take a nap or a shower *in the middle of the day.* Yes, you read that right...in the middle of the day. Tell me, my friend...what nurse gets to do that??

Now let's compare this to floor nursing and count the ways it's better, shall we?

Or better yet, maybe I could tell you what I miss about my old job at the PACU...hmmm, it's a tough one, really...maybe it's the morning commute and all the traffic. Or maybe it's having a patient scream at me after coming off of anesthesia because he (or she) feels crappy, and somehow, that's all the nurse's fault. Or maybe it's being on my feet for crazy, long 12 hour shifts and needing orthopedic shoes because my feet were always somewhere between agony-level pain or totally numb at the end of the day. Or, I've got a good one...maybe it's the office politics that have no place in a medical setting, but you and I both know they're there, and we can either play along, or find ourselves out of a job.

But here's the really great thing about Marie...and I promise it's another thing that might make you think she's at least partially divine...it's not just her amazing program that provides the requisite experience that's required to get these work from home nursing jobs. It's not even all the things you'll learn from the program itself. It's that she helped me put together a killer resume that would get noticed by potential employers. It's that she taught me how to interview like a champ. And the cherry on top is that she actually lists job opportunities like an insider guru job board. She's like one of those one stop shops for everything you need to make a lot of money working from home as a nurse, all the while still being a healer and an advocate for patients.

Let me end this with a story (within a story, haha!) because this story may be all you need to understand why you need Marie.

So, I had an interview for a chronic care manager position. It was set up as a Zoom call because you know, Covid. Well, get this...my camera worked like a dream a few days before the interview, when I tested it...because we nurses always prepare, right? But then, as luck would have it, my camera somehow did NOT work on the day of the interview. So the interviewer agreed to stick to audio only. And then my audio crashes right in the middle of the interview.

Now remember, I'm a nurse, not a tech guru, so my attempts to fix the problem did not bear any fruit. We ended up finishing the interview over our cell phones...and in spite of all that, I still got a job offer! And you know why? Because Marie taught me every last thing I needed to know, so that I wouldn't sweat it, even when everything seemed to be going wrong. I was so confident that I was the best candidate for the job that nothing and no one could shake me.

So let me put it to you like this...if you're a nurse and you're ready to make some serious impact AND some serious money without having to get up off your sofa, you need Marie Peppers. Thank me later...I promise that you'll want to.

Lisa Brooks, RN

MICHELLE'S STORY

I always knew I wanted to be a nurse. Don't get me wrong, I realize I'm not the only little girl who pretended to be a nurse when I was playing.

But for me it was something deeper than just a game of Florence Nightingale. It was a calling; something deep in my soul longing to come out and be fulfilled.

I started nurturing that dream by becoming a candy striper in high school. Believe it or not, I still have the uniform in my closet. But life has a way of knocking you around a bit; it's not the straight path we were led to believe it is, back when we were children, goofing around with a plastic stethoscope and an Operation game, trying hard not to set off the buzzer.

So I went into accounting instead. And let's be honest, it's a safer path. Numbers don't die on you, they don't vomit on you, and they don't have family members grieving their loss. I don't know if I can even tell you for sure why I initially abandoned the nursing path for accounting. Maybe some part of me was afraid of the emotional toll of being a nurse. Maybe another part of me just saw accounting as an easier path.

But dreams die hard, don't they? And my dream was no exception. The desire to be a nurse couldn't be counted away, no matter how many numbers I crunched.So I enrolled in an LPN program, and then got my Bachelor's of Science in 2004. Well, that's how it started, anyway.

Now let's talk a bit about how it's going....

See, Covid hit, and it altered my reality. Not just because as a nurse, I was an essential worker expected to risk my life at every turn, no questions asked. Not because nursing became any more difficult, at least not in the usual sense of more patients filling wards, and more people struggling to breathe without a ventilator. I mean, sure, those things were issues, no question about it.

But for me, the problem was bigger than that. You see, I was born with significant hearing loss, and despite my parents' best efforts, along with countless trips to doctors and specialists, nothing could be done about it, other than handing me a pair of bulky, awkward hearing aids that spent much of my childhood hidden in my pockets. Not much good they did me in there.

The thing about not being able to hear is that you learn to read lips, and you become exceptionally good at it. If we're honest, a better way to say it is...you learn to completely rely on it.

But mask mandates have a way of complicating that because I could no longer see anyone's lips. And suddenly, I had no idea what was being said to me, what was being said around me, and what my patients truly needed. Imagine all of this happening in the midst of a pandemic where there was already a sense of panic and despair in the air. I knew something had to change.

Some might have told me that this would have been the perfect moment to hang up my scrubs for good and get back into the accounting game. But I couldn't do that because underneath it all, I have the heart and soul of a nurse, and I wasn't going to give up so easily.

Some things are meant to be, just like I was meant to go into nursing. And ultimately, the Universe always has a way of putting the right people in our path, just when we need them. All we have to do is follow our instincts and meet them halfway. That's when I heard about Marie Peppers.

So, here's the thing about Marie...she, too, is a nurse. Unlike me, her hearing is just fine. But she quickly figured out something that so many others didn't even notice...that there are SO many ways to be of service and help people as a nurse. And they don't all involve risking our lives in the middle of a modern plague. They certainly don't all require people like me to struggle to do my job where lives are on the line, simply because I wasn't able to hear what's going on around me, or what was being said directly to me.

At the risk of sounding a bit dramatic, Marie's programs have saved my life, my career, and my sanity. But in more practical terms, she's simply altered my reality by making my childhood dream possible, even under the worst of circumstances, even with a hearing impairment (for which insurance won't cover the cost of solutions because they don't consider hearing necessary to be a nurse!), and the very best part...I can be a nurse without having to leave my home.

In practical terms, that means I still get to save lives without masks, without risks, without the struggle, and without having to be reminded all the time that I can't hear what everyone else hears; a struggle that most employers (and busy hospital administrators) can't even begin to fathom.

Whereas many people grumbled at the inconvenience of having to wear a mask, for me, it literally ended my career as a bedside nurse. My girlhood dream, starting from when I could talk, leading to being a candy striper in high school, and ultimately sending me into a whirlwind of hospital codes, and being an angel for people who were scared and hurting could have died right there. But thanks to Marie, it didn't, and it won't. Working as a nurse from my home means I can do this well past the age of retirement if I want to continue to do so, without any of the downsides of being on my feet for 12 hour shifts day after day after day.

Let's be honest here...nursing is not glamorous. And if you're in it for the money, my best advice is to find a new career. If you don't have a nurse's heart, no amount of money will get you through a stillbirth (and the devastated family affected by it), a patient dying (and once again, the devastated family affected by it), or just the simple daily task of having sick patients vomit or poop on you.

But if you truly want to save lives and leave this world better than it was when you came into it, nursing is one of the best and most rewarding ways to do that.

And if being able to do it from home sounds appealing; showing up daily from the comfort of your home office for companies that rely on you to make exceptional patient care possible, then there's no one better than Marie Peppers to show you how to do that. I still get the benefit of building lasting relationships. I still get to save lives. I still get to make a difference. I still get to be an important cog (however small each of us may be in this wheel) in a wheel that needs to turn every day in order to make life livable for humans in our society. And in the world of nursing, no job is too small or insignificant. We are ultimately the ones patients rely on. We are the ones who make each patient's care seamless and as comfortable as possible, we are the ones who patients will remember long after we've moved on to the next patient.

So make no mistake...you don't have to be a martyr on a hospital floor to be a nurse. You CAN do an amazing job and still change the world without leaving your home. And with Marie's help, you can meet other amazing nurses and make friendships along the way that will last you a lifetime. If I found my way here because a mask mandate made my day to day job impossible, and in the process, discovered the most amazing and happiest way to make use of my years of education and on the floor training, then what's stopping you...?

Michelle Niccum, RN

VIVIEN'S STORY

S o, I may as well just lead with it...I'm The oddball here.

What I mean is that I am not a nurse.

Now, don't get me wrong, I was a pharmacist for many years, I even had my own pharmacy in my native Australia...and then I came to the US and worked in the medical sales business...so it's not as if I'm a stranger to all things medical.

But, as I said, I am the oddball here because, alas, I am not a nurse.

So, why is my story here, you ask, in a compilation book of nurses' stories?

Well, I'm glad you asked!

Everything comes down to Marie Peppers...and when I say "everything," in this case, I really do mean *everything*. She didn't just put together an amazing program...on top of that, Marie hosts retreats for her nurses, and she asked me to come and speak at them, in order to teach, coach, and most of all, inspire.

Maybe it sounds cliche (these days, anyway), but I gave up my old career to become a life coach. And no, it's not a decision I made lightly, nor did I choose this because it's in vogue nowadays.

The thing is that I was raised by hardworking, high-achieving parents, who moved from Holland to Australia with only a tiny suitcase filled with their worldly belongings, a hope, a prayer, grit, and determination to succeed. And that's the attitude I was raised in...if you're not overachieving, then are you even achieving anything at all?

What I learned, though, is that one can be an overachiever, and not a high achiever at the same time. It's a conundrum, I know, but bear with me.

I lived in a world where I was busy with something every moment I was awake, simply because otherwise I'd have idle hands, and we all know whose work they do, right? And I don't even mean this in a religious sense. At all. It was about always having something to show for every minute of my time. But underneath it all, I was missing the point of life...following my passions, fulfilling my purpose, and most of all, going forward without fear...or as I like to put it, moving through my discomfort zone because everything I want is in that zone, and I've had to be willing to get uncomfortable to get it.

So let me simplify it a bit...there's a beautiful hike near where I live...and there are two ways to get there. The first one is the easy way...you drive your car up to the top, and then you hike around up at the top.

Or, you can walk the whole way, starting at the bottom, making your way to the top, and then hike back down the mountain...it's a rough and tumble 12 miles.

We all know which way sounds easiest, but it misses out on a huge dopamine boost...the reward of making the treacherous climb, managing to miss all the gnarly roots and other elements of nature in our paths, just waiting to trip us and bring us down. The drive sort of misses the point, but it's popular with people who want to get to the top without doing the work.

In life, you don't get to do that, though. The work, the obstacles, the hurdles, the fears and dangers that lurk in your discomfort zone are the ripe environment where you grow your best self, claw your way out of your old self that no longer serves you, and let go of all the limiting beliefs that have been holding you back.

Why am I telling you all this, you ask?

Because I get it. Nursing is HARD. Changing the way you do nursing is daunting. Taking more classes can be terrifying. And there's that good, old-fashioned fear of the unknown.

Yes, bedside nursing wreaks havoc on your body. Hospital politics are pure hell. 12 hour shifts (that easily turn into 15 hour shifts) are exhausting.

But at least it's the devil you know, right?

Here's what I want to tell you (and this is the main reason I'm here)...you don't have to settle for any devil...there IS a better way, even if you have to venture outside your comfort zone to get it. And I get the stress of taking classes while still carrying out your job, taking care of your kiddos, and simply keeping your house clean (and yourself sane!) is a huge burden. But it's a journey through your discomfort zone, and it's sort of like the magic in "Alice in Wonderland," because once you take the plunge and dive into that rabbithole, Wonderland is on the other side of it.

And if you're nervous, or simply think you can't do it, that you're going to be that one statistic in Marie's world who did not land an amazing job after finishing her program, I'm here to coach you through that, help you de-stress, and show you how powerful and amazing you truly are.

Let me close this out by sharing my three core values that you get you up that mountain...because life is a proverbial hike, and if you're only willing to drive to the top, keep it safe, meander around at the top a bit, and then hop back in your car and head home, then your rewards will be minimal, just as your risk and effort were minimal. But if you're willing to take a deep breath, prepare your body for a lengthy (and sometimes painful) journey, then the rewards waiting for you at the top of that mountain are immense beyond words.

So let's dig into those three things, shall we?

Without further ado, they are....

1. Self belief. Plainly stated, you have to believe you can do it. And a huge part of that is simply acknowledging where you currently are, and where you want to go...what does the finish line look like? Who do you have to be to get there?

2. Courage. Taking on a new project, and in this case, pivoting the way you go about nursing takes courage. Any change brings discomfort, and that alone takes courage. Without self belief, though, there is no courage, so this stems from core value number 1.

3. Action. Just wanting it is not enough. Just believing it's possible, or that you can do it, or that you'll be great at is not enough. Dreams are good, but if you don't act on them, they'll forever remain dreams and nothing more.

So, bottom line..if you believe in yourself (and you should because nurses are true healers and world changers!), if you have the courage (if you didn't, you'd not have chosen nursing as a career), and if you're ready to take action to completely change your life for the better, then sign up for Marie's program.

And if you're struggling, I'm here to coach you through the journey. I believe in you already, and Marie does, too. So what are you waiting for?

Vivien Hudson - The Stress & Performance Coach

WHAT'S NEXT?

So now you know all about the possibilities available to you RIGHT NOW!

No more 12+ hour shifts on your feet...if you don't want to.

No more driving through crazy traffic to get to work...if you don't want to.

No more playing political games at work...if you don't want to.

No more leaving your family on Christmas Day to work...well, you get it.

Do you want to?

Want to know HOW to live like the nurses in these stories...?

And you know what else?

There are TONS of remote work opportunities in Case-Care Management for RNs and LPNs!

So, you read all about the ways my course changed those nurses' lives in radical and amazing ways...and I get it, you want some of that for yourself. I don't blame you a bit.

My course is one way you can achieve remote ready skills.

Another option is getting on-the-job training at a facility. Many facilities want you to work in their building if they decide to give you training.

My course was tailor-made to teach you the skills you need to succeed working remote from home.

Now, let's be clear here...my course is **not required** for you to work from home as a nurse...it's not like those prerequisites you had to take in college...we're not back in school in that way.

BUT...

You can do this the easy way by taking my course that will walk you through the entire process.

Or you can do it the hard way by trying to figure it all out for yourself.

You decide, Nurse.

I know you're curious, so let me give you a few details on this course:

1. I've been teaching it for just over 3 years now. And it's constantly evolving with new information as more remote work becomes available for nurses like you.

2. I have a team of 5 RNs and 4 LPNs who assist me with our online teaching services for nurses.

3. To qualify, you need to be a nurse with a minimum of one year bedside clinical experience...seriously...that's all you need to make this happen and live your dream life as a nurse.

And what we offer is...drumroll, please....

Remote Learning Services, LLC
Care/Case Management, Remote Patient Monitoring, HEDIS Data Abstracting and Wellness Coaching, THE 4-in-1 program (Certificate program)

We also offer Utilization Review 101 for RNs and LPNs - Certificate program

Coming soon in 2023 (2 new mini courses)
- Diabetic Nutritional Nurse-Health Coach, Certificate program

-Telephonic Triage Careers for Registered Nurses, Certificate program

Find my **courses** on the Teachable platform
https://chronic-care-manager-course-medicare-
ccm.teachable.com/courses

One thing I'd like to add is that in truly healer fashion, I really want to help and guide nurses, even if you're not interested in taking my program. I'm always here to offer nurses guidance, especially newly minted nurses...I know how excited but also, overwhelmed and sometimes, downright shell-shocked you're feeling because I've been where you are, and I still remember. Feel free to reach out to me...I'm here for you, whether you enter my program or not.

Follow Marie on Linkedin - Remote Nurse Jobs https://www.linkedin.com/in/remotenursejobs

Marie is working with Senior Corporate Clinical Recruiters for Molina Healthcare and many other major employers. Check her often to see what jobs she may share.

Join my **Facebook group Community** of 33K nurses at **Remote Nursing Jobs Work-From-Home, RN/LPN by Remote Learning LLC**

Hope to see you there.

Because I've been where you are, and I know how hard it is.

I also know how much easier and more rewarding it can be...and I can help you get there...are you ready for this?

Made in United States
North Haven, CT
29 January 2024

48037880R00046